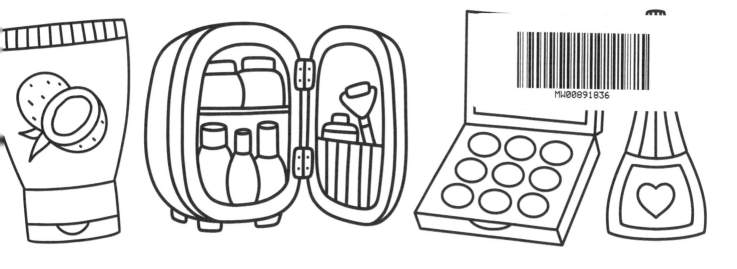

COSMETICS
Easy Coloring Book

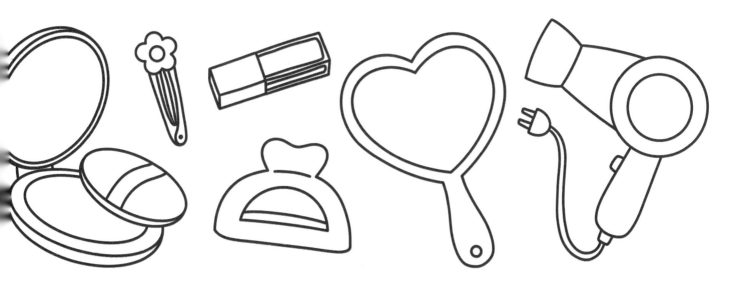

MW00891836

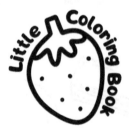

Copyright © 2024 Little Coloring Book

Cosmetics Easy Coloring Book: Cute & Simple Illustrations for All Ages

ISBN: 9798324816162

The designs in this volume are intended for personal use of the reader and may not be reproduced.

Hi there!

Thank you so much for picking up one of my easy coloring books! I appreciate all the love and support! :)

Just a friendly reminder that even though the pages are single-sided, you'll still need to place a thick paper or cardstock underneath when using markers to prevent any bleed-through. This little trick will keep your coloring book neat and beautiful.

Happy coloring!

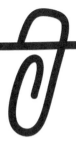

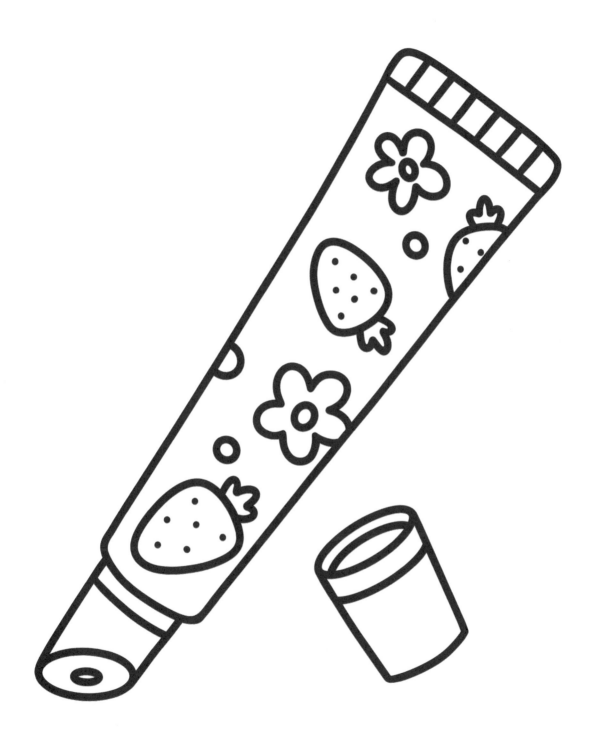

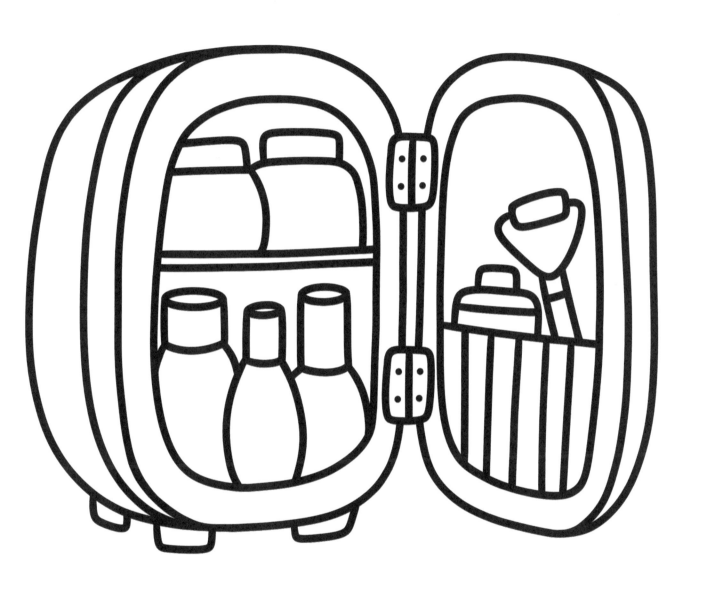

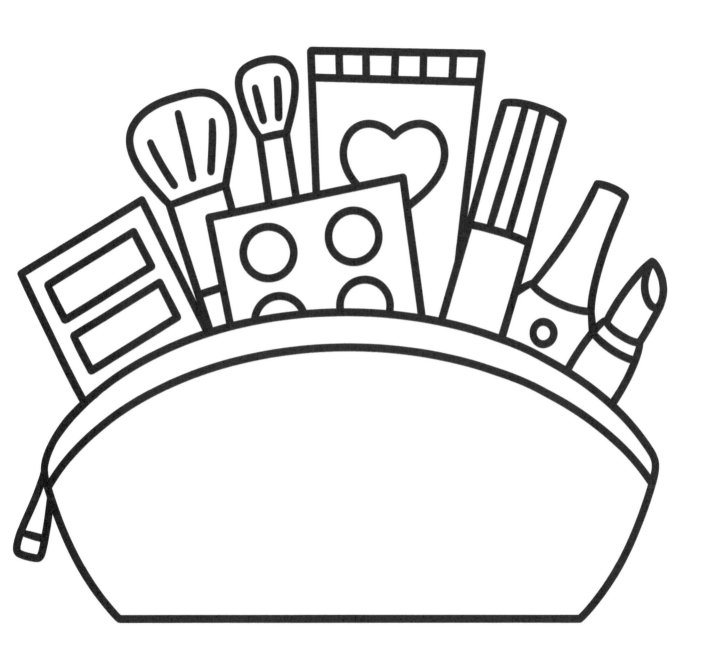

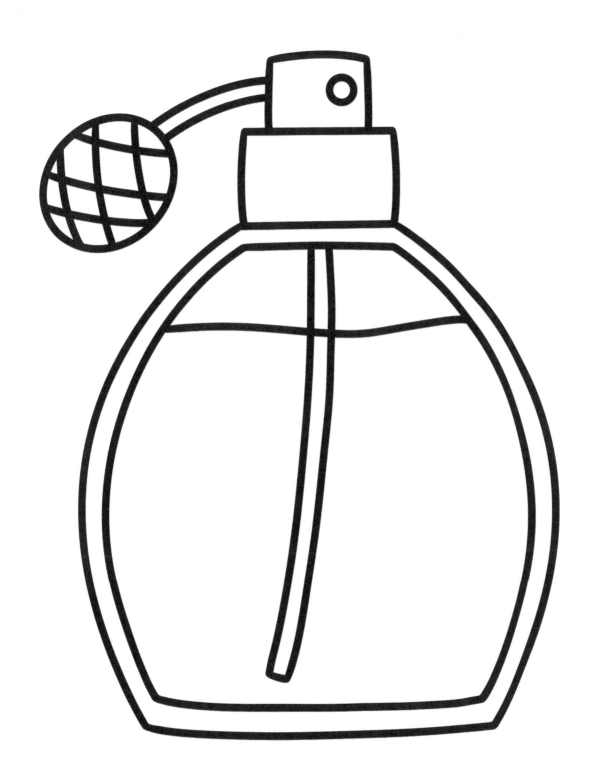

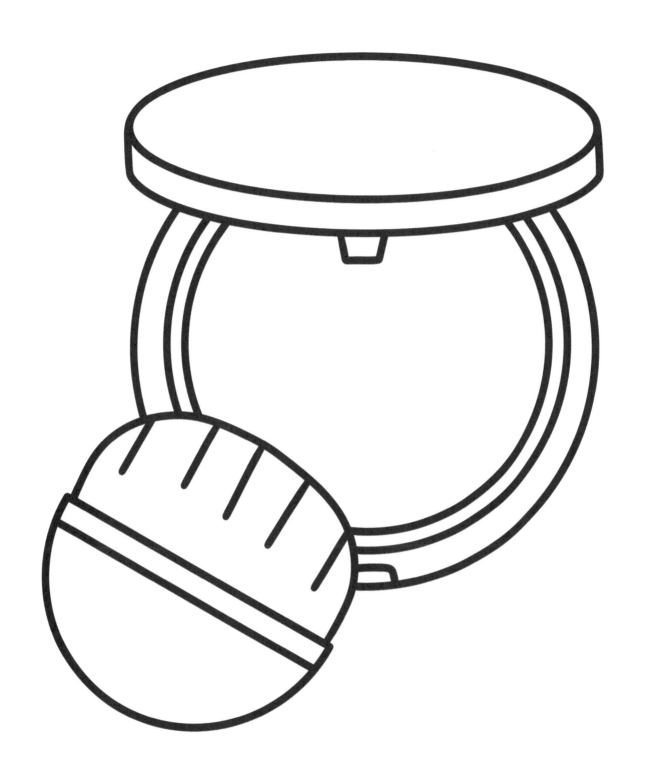

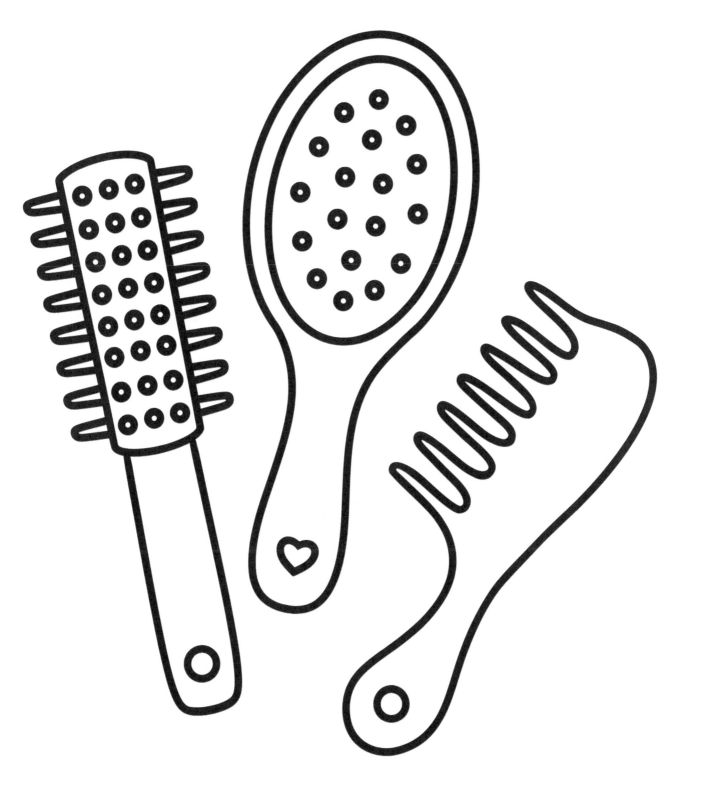

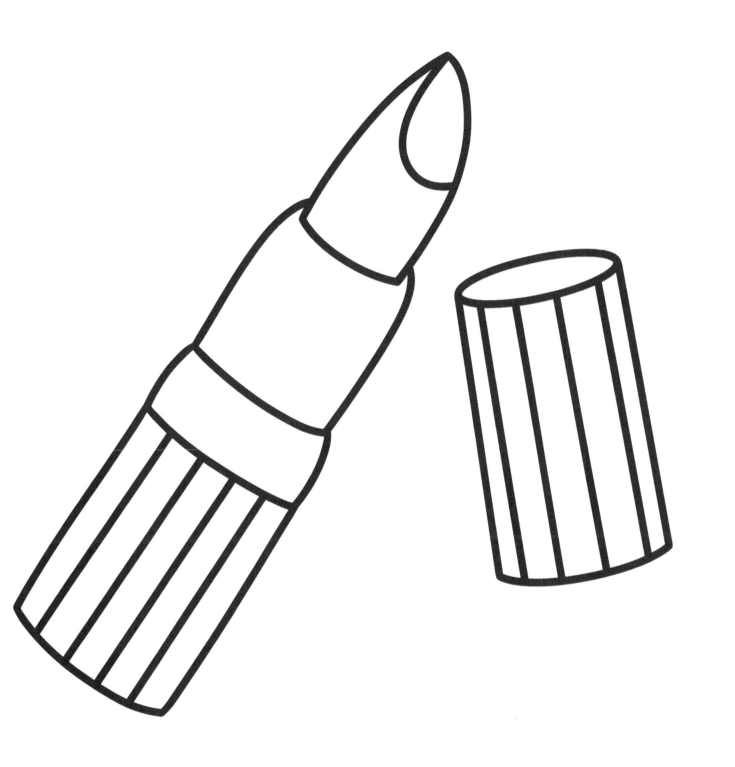

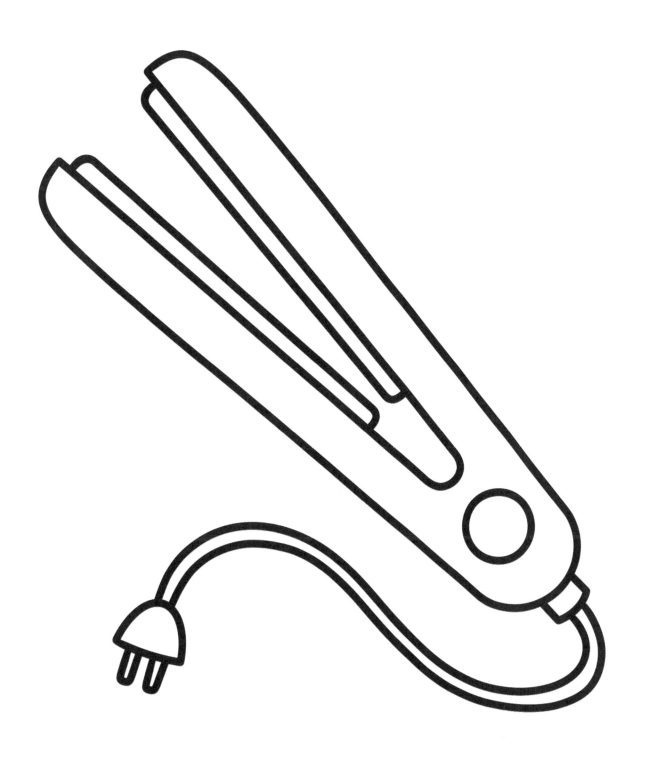

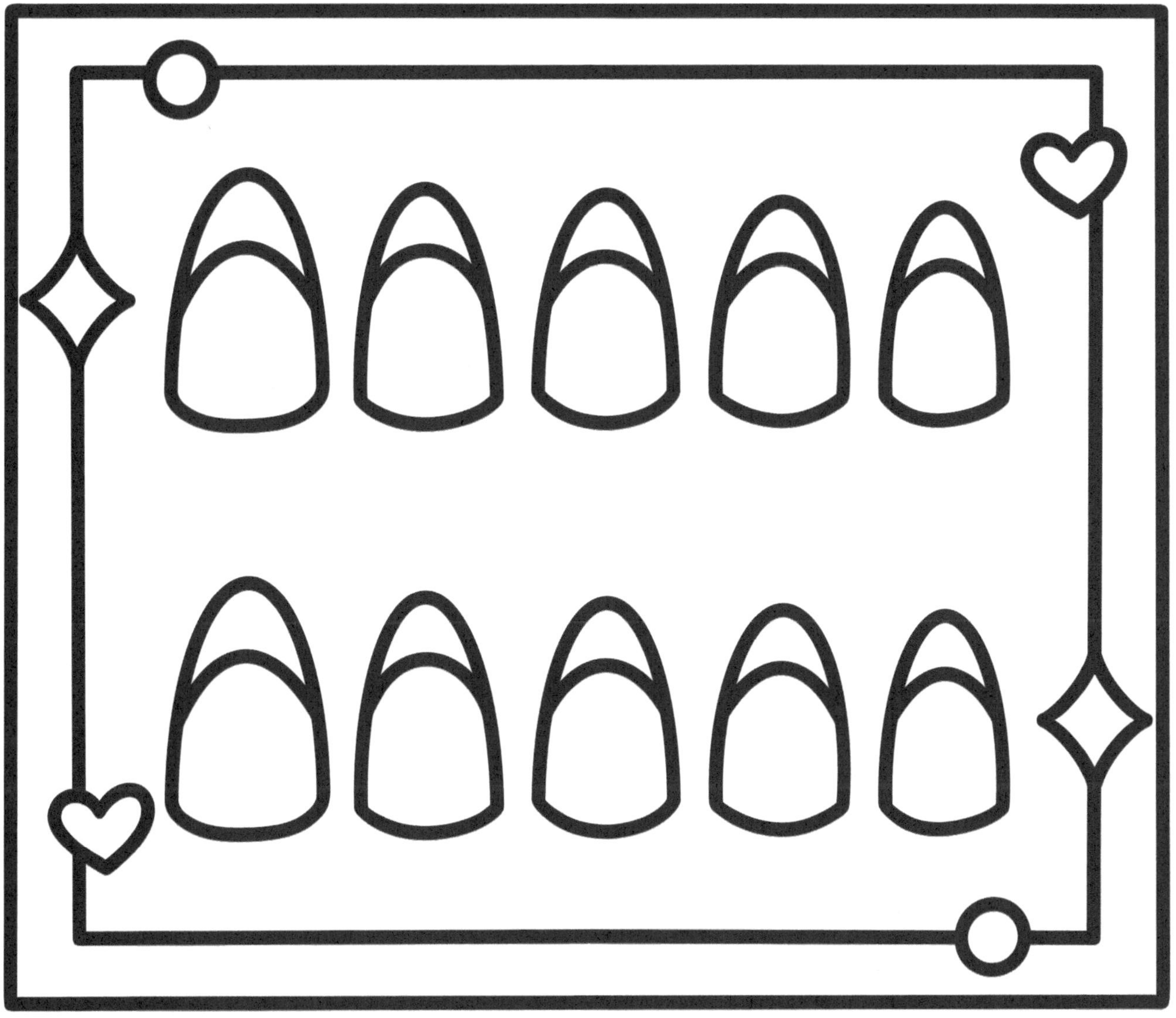

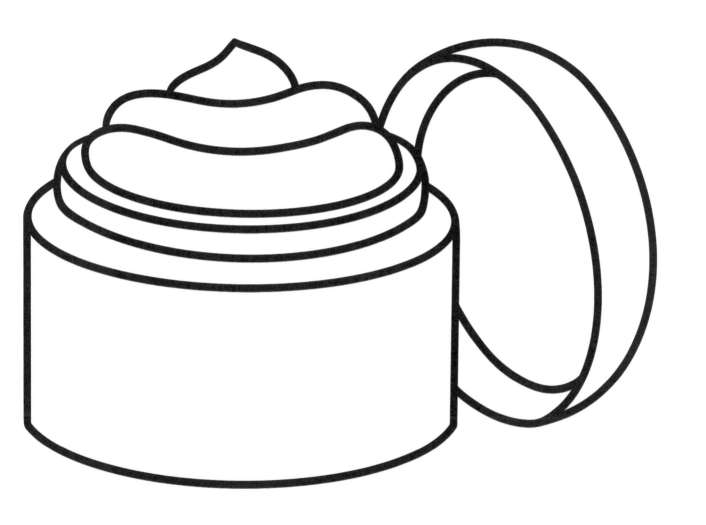

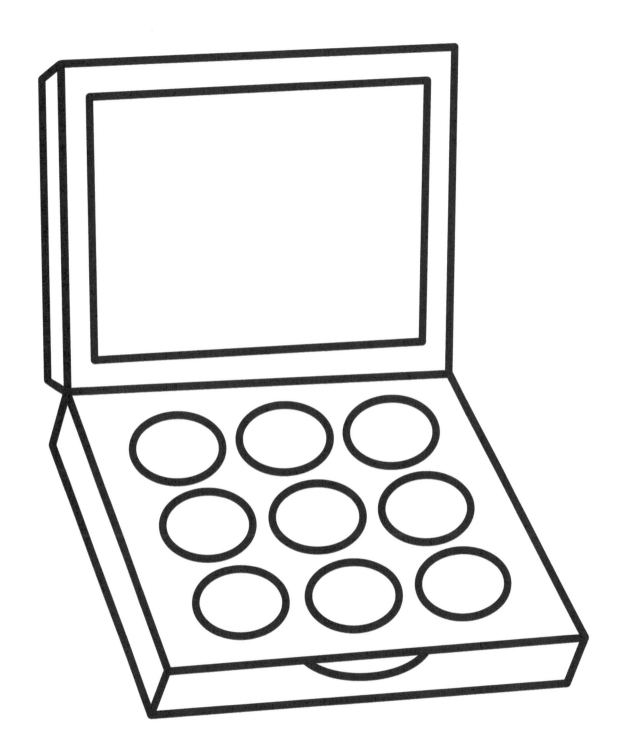

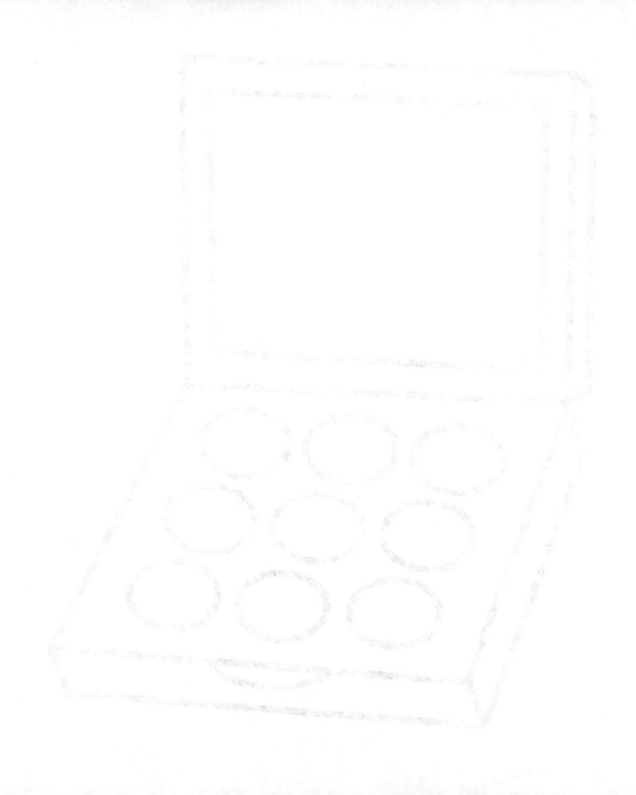

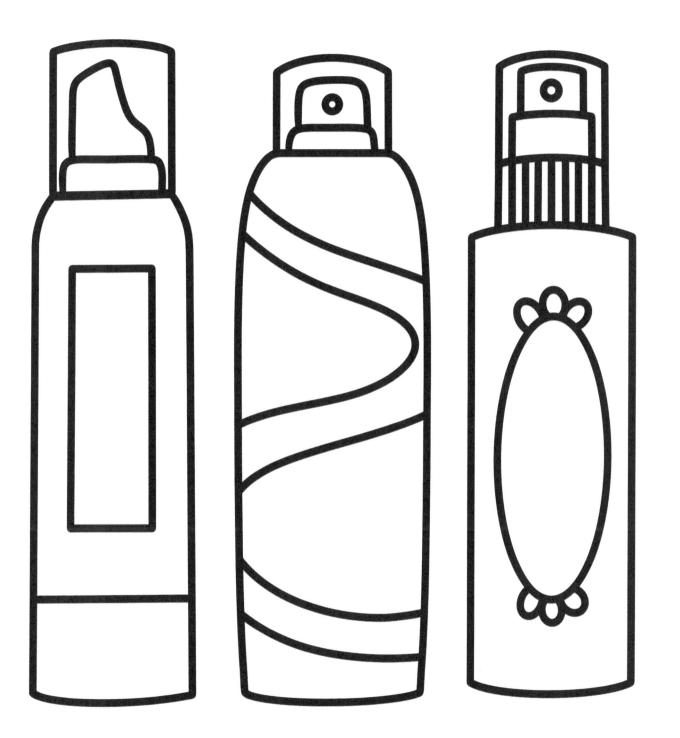

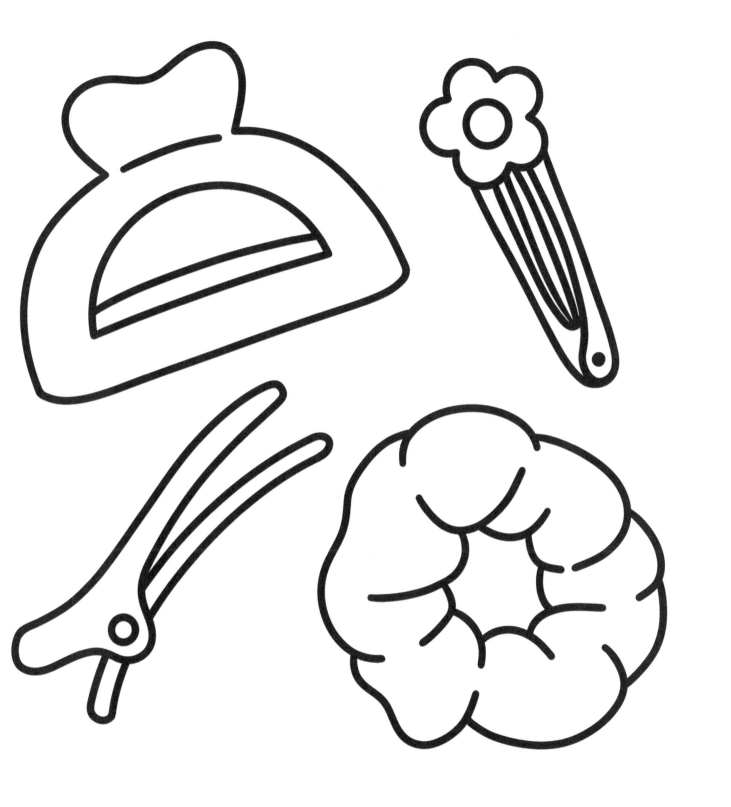

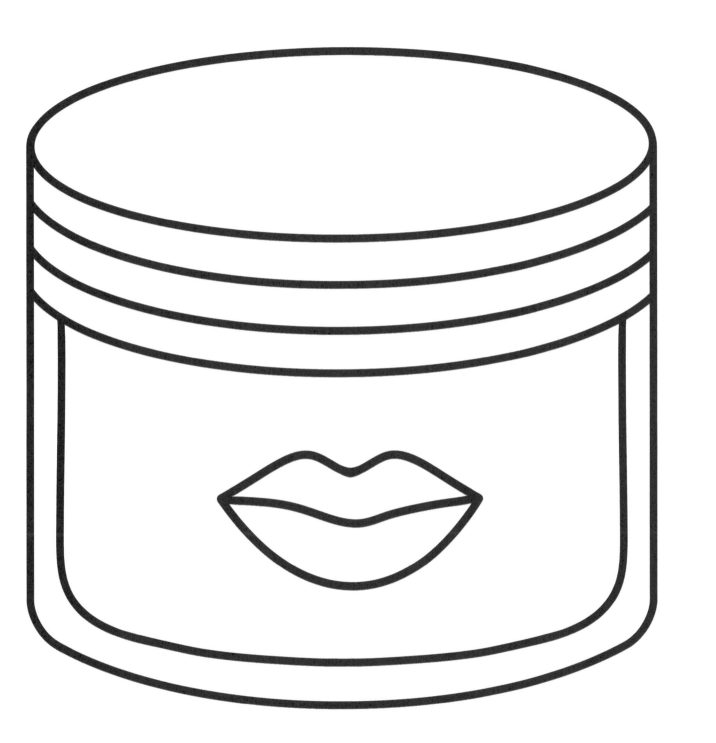

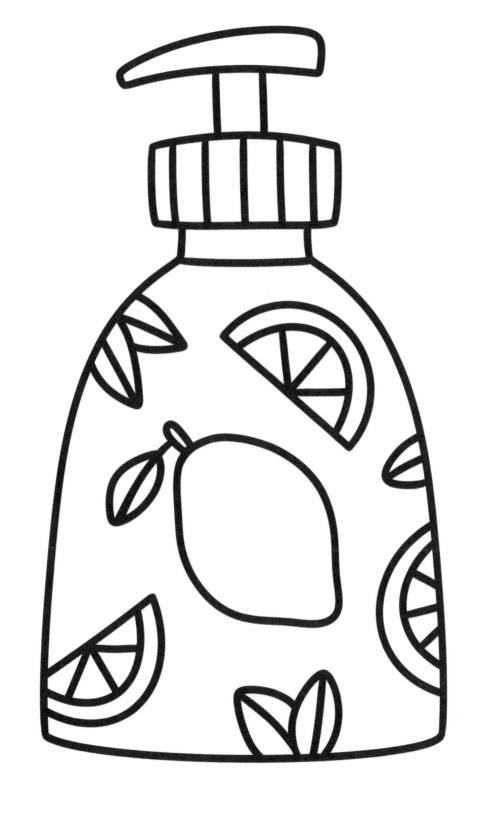

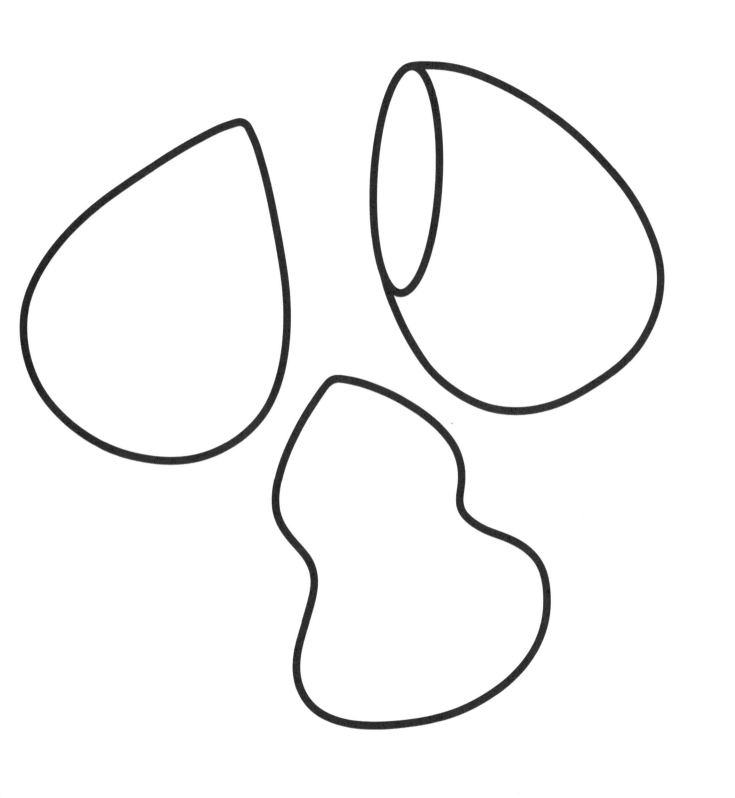

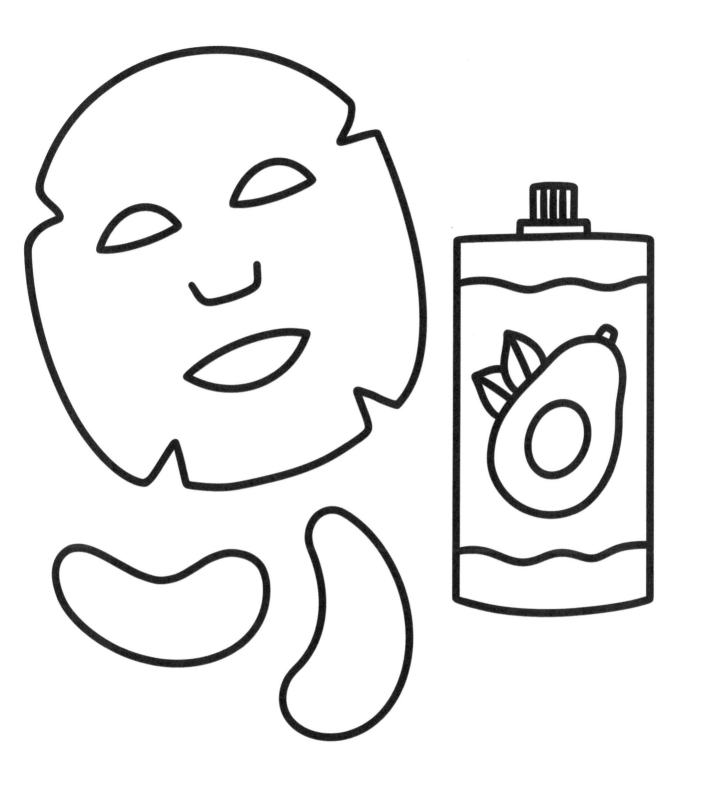

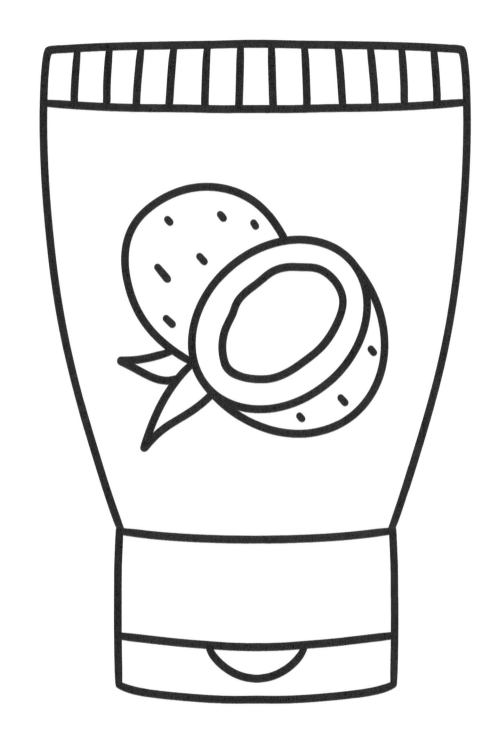

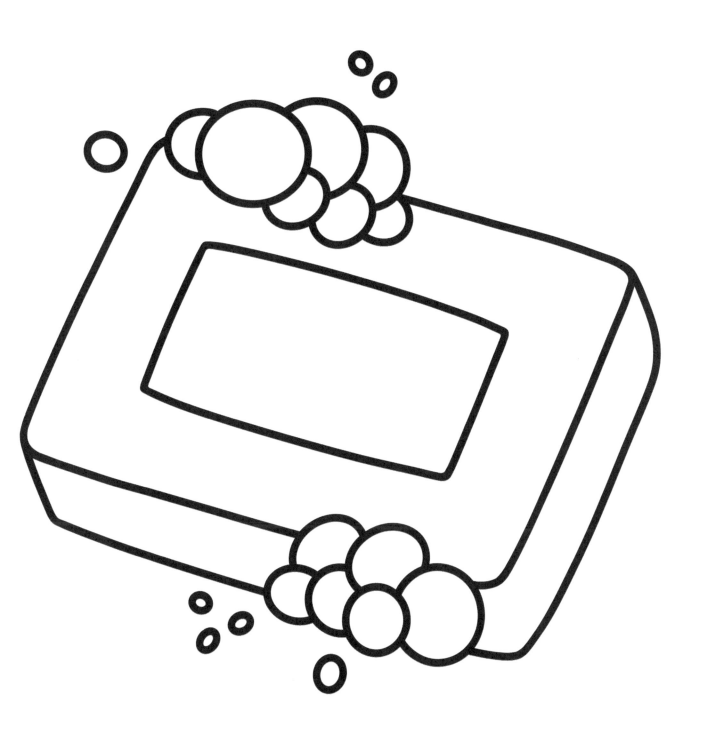

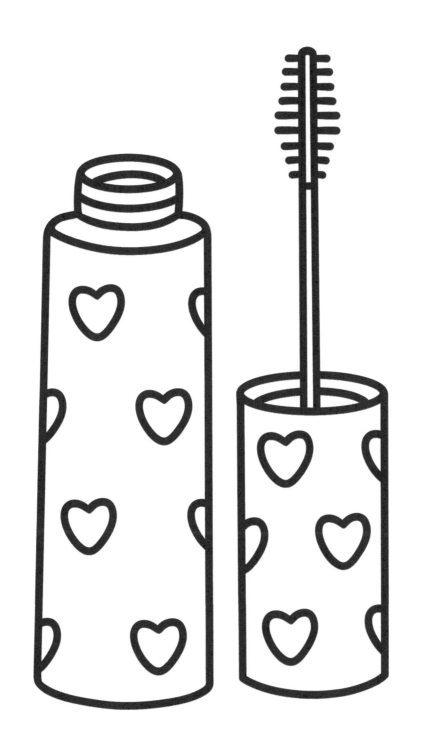

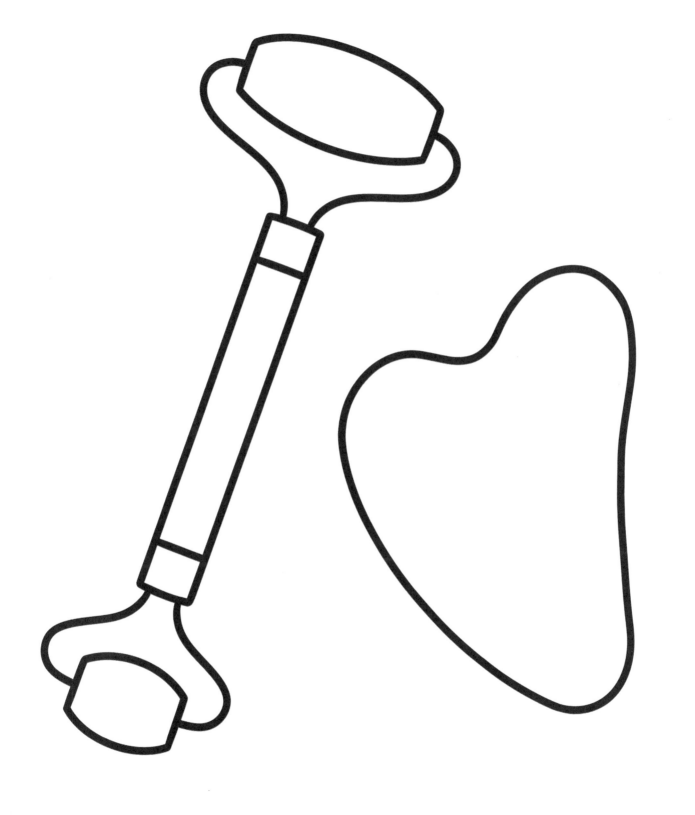

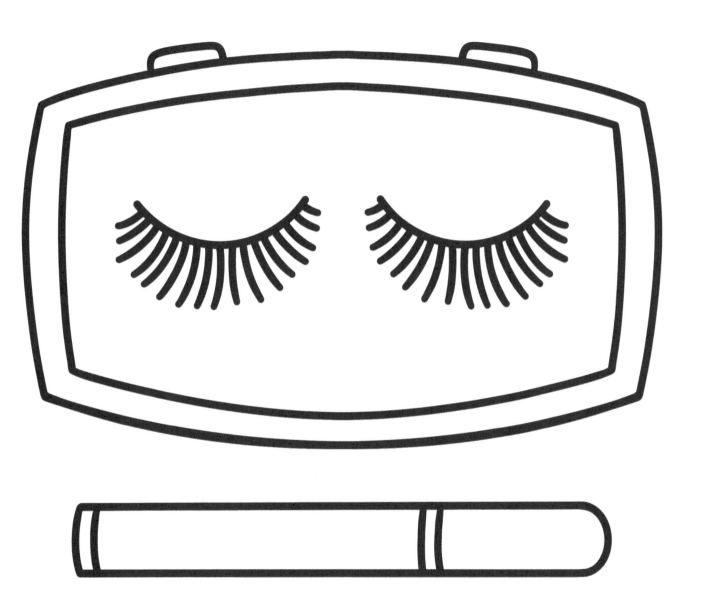

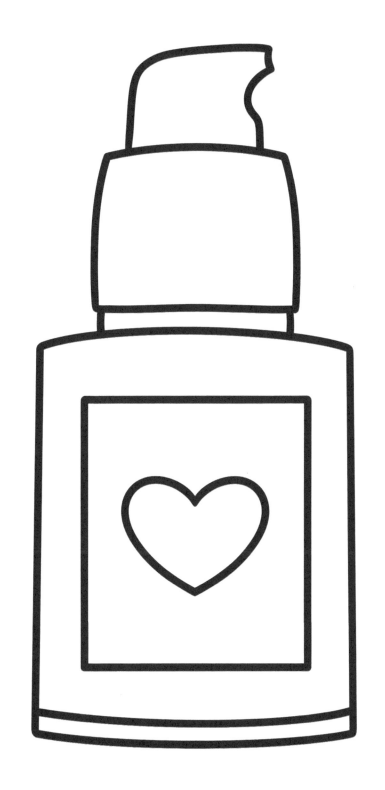

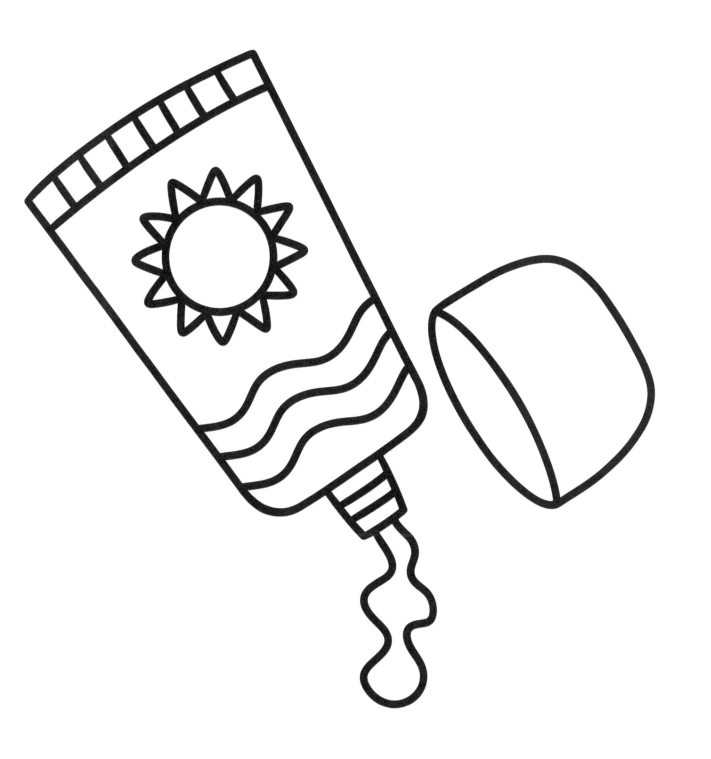

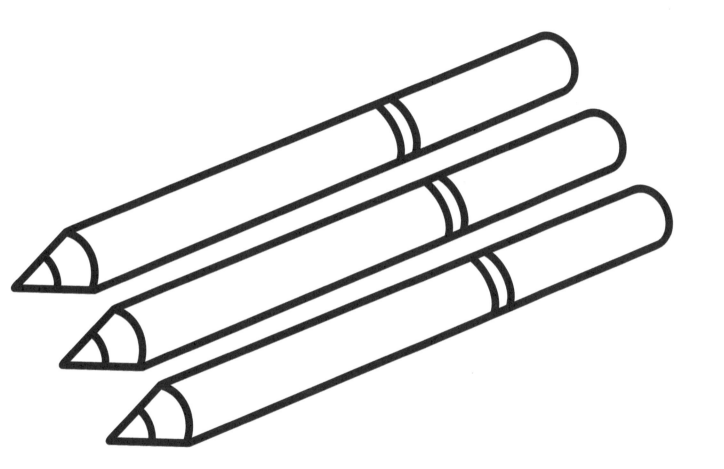

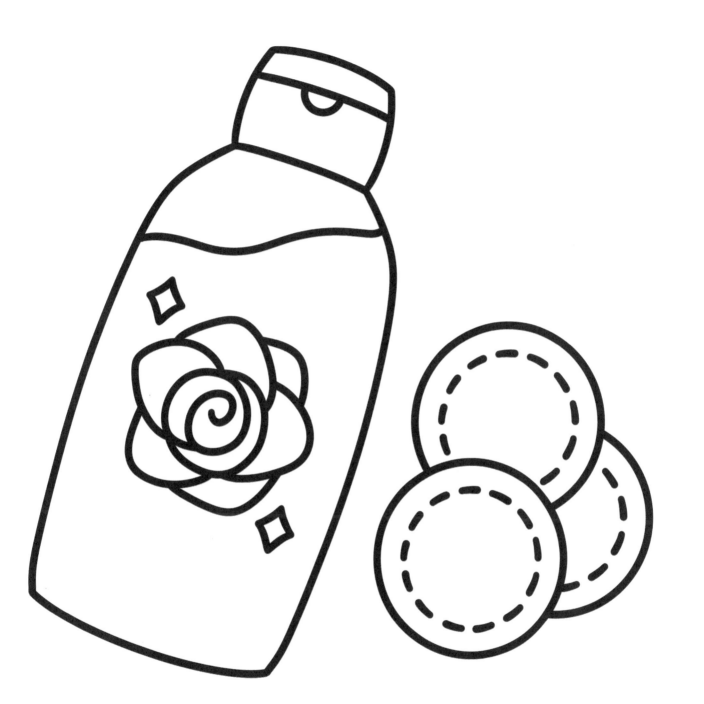

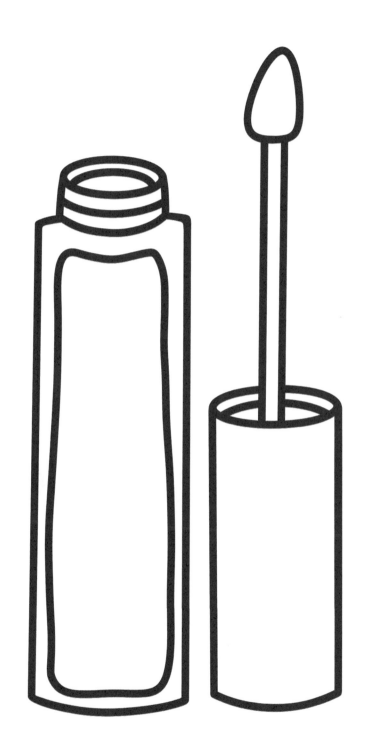

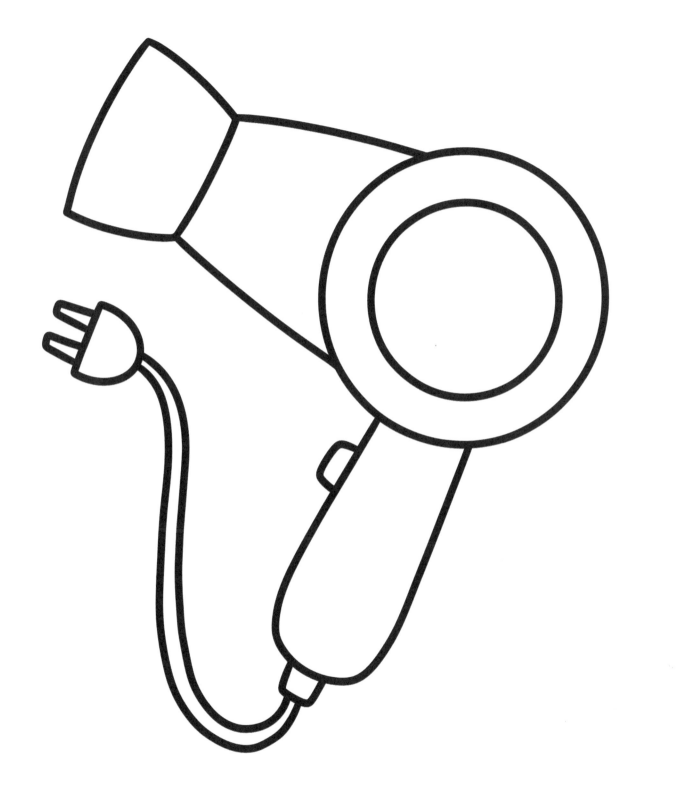

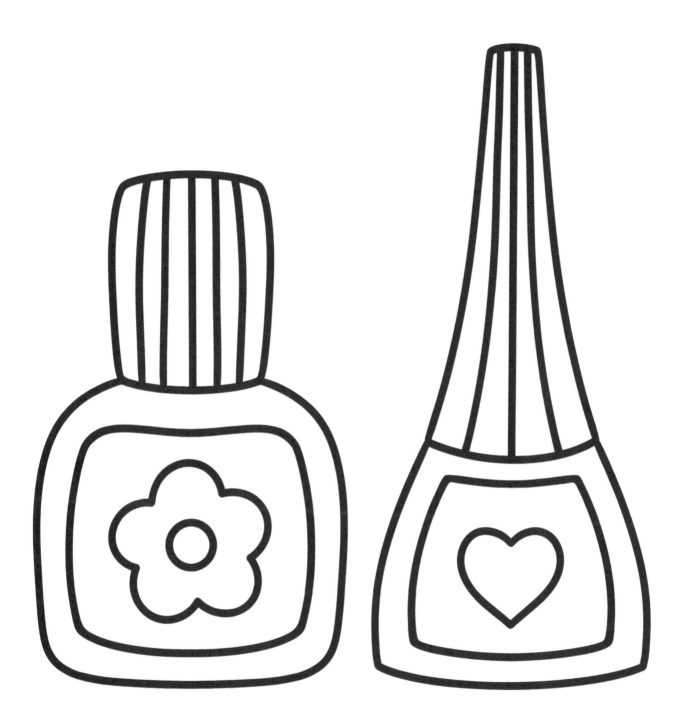

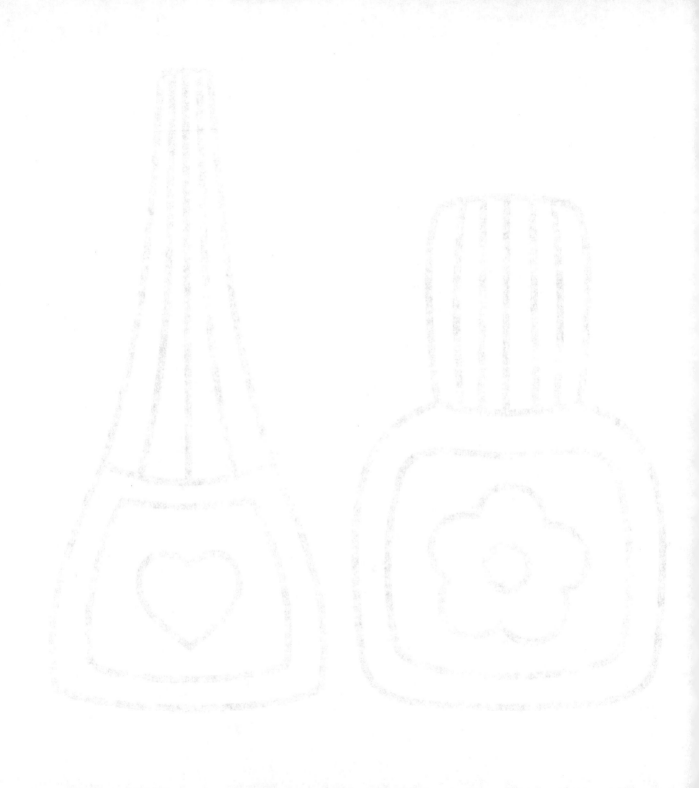

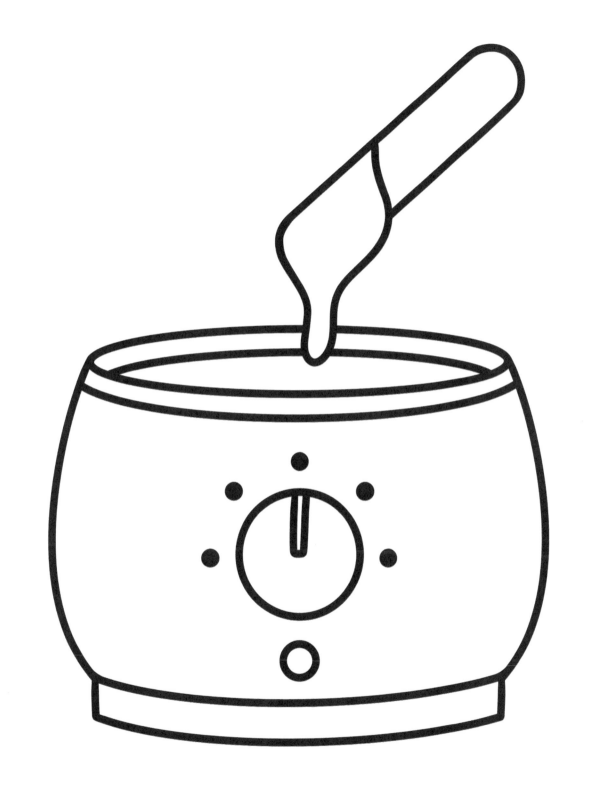

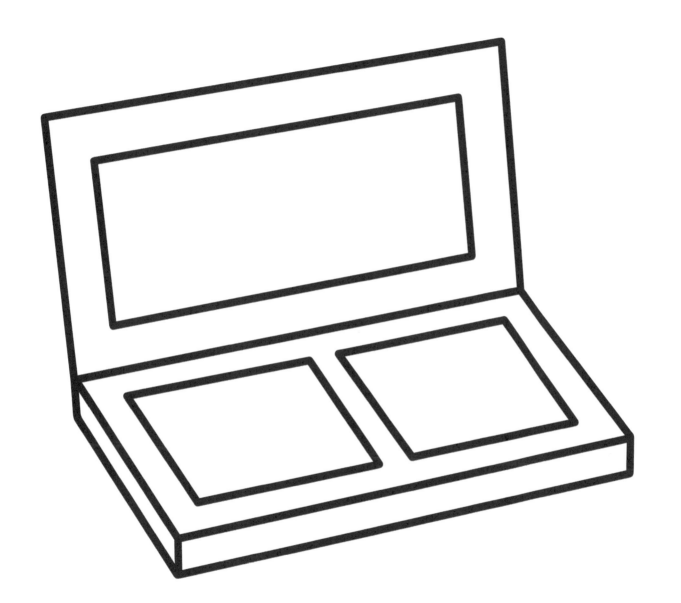

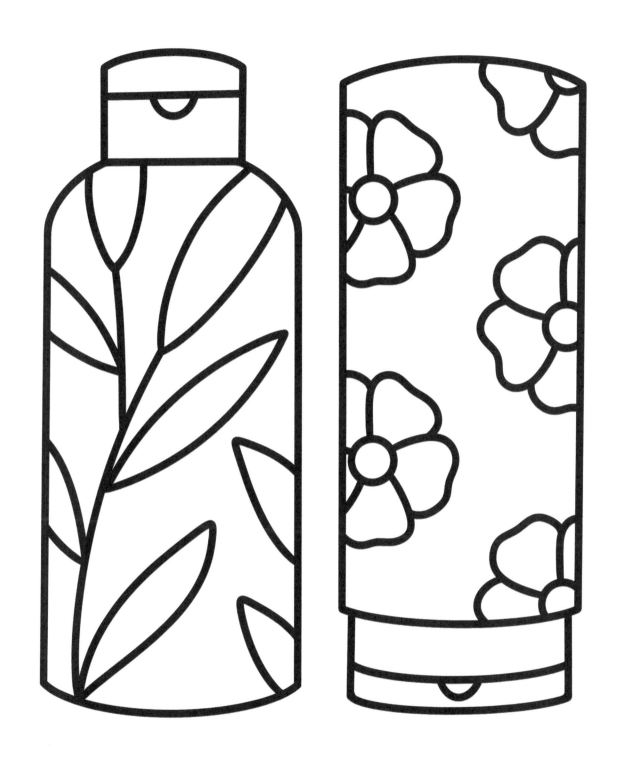

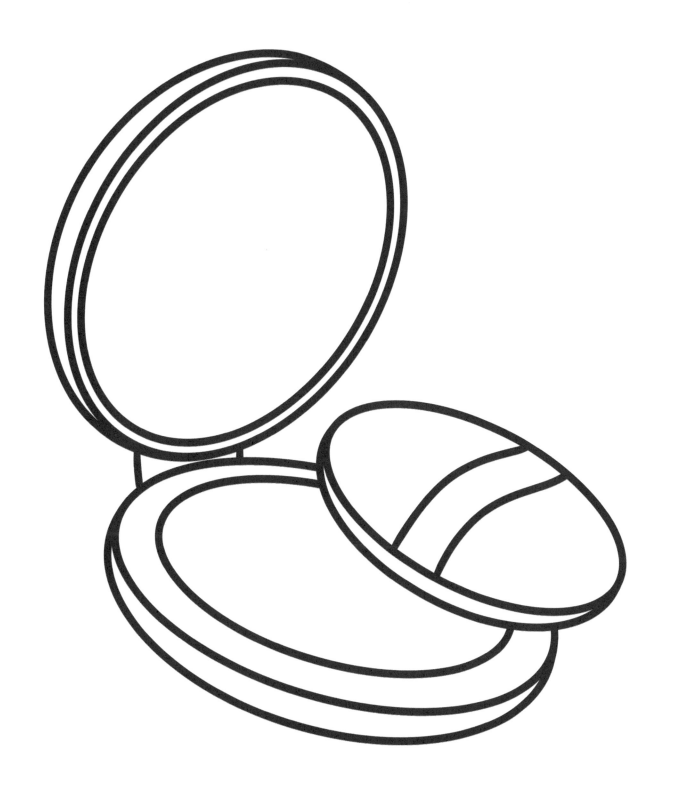

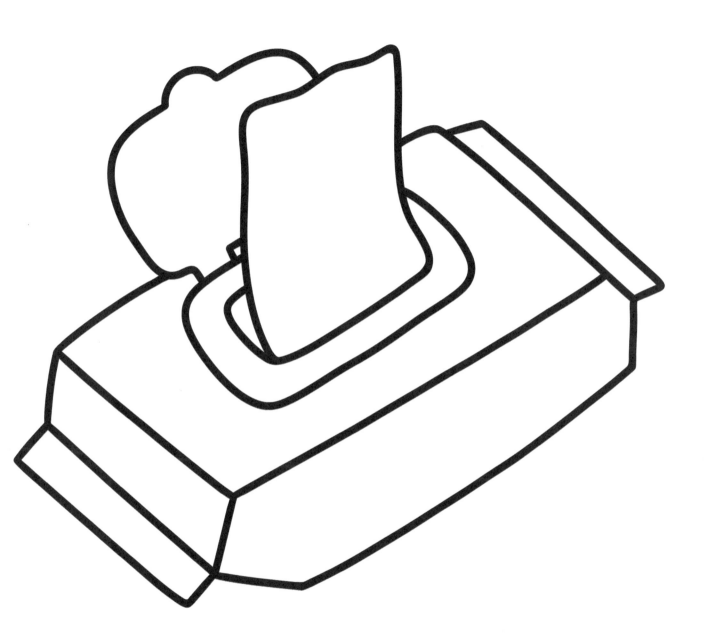

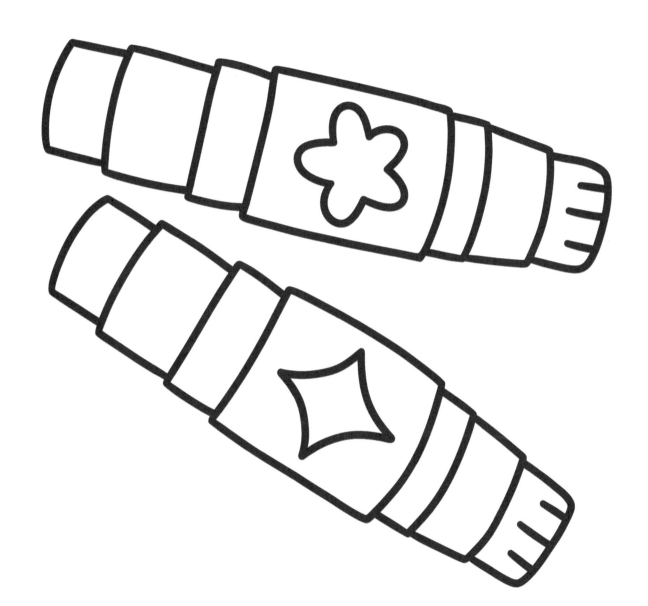

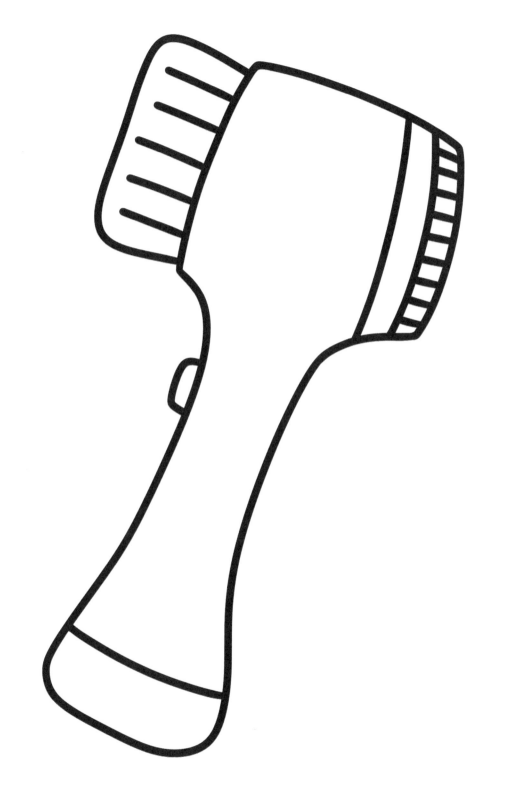

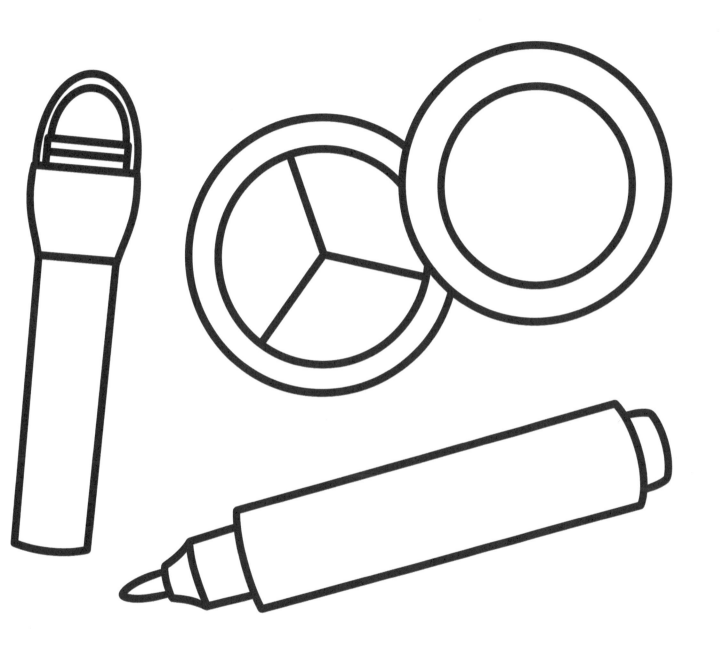

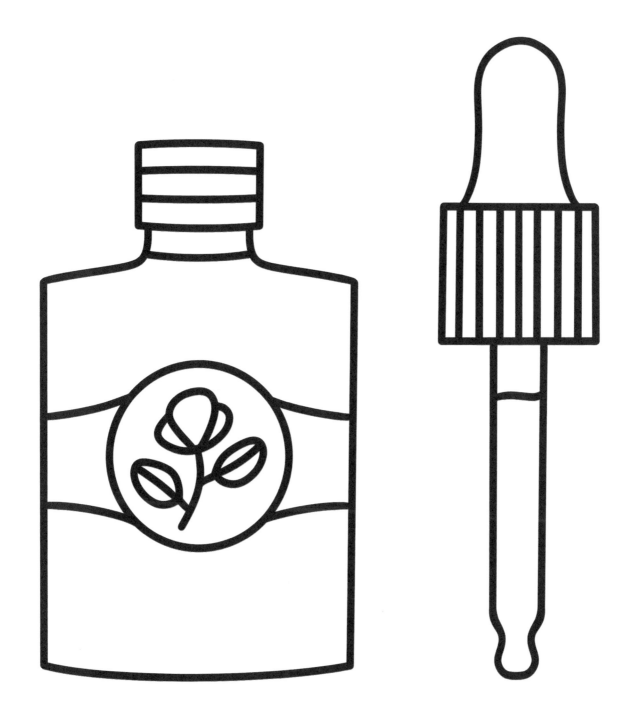

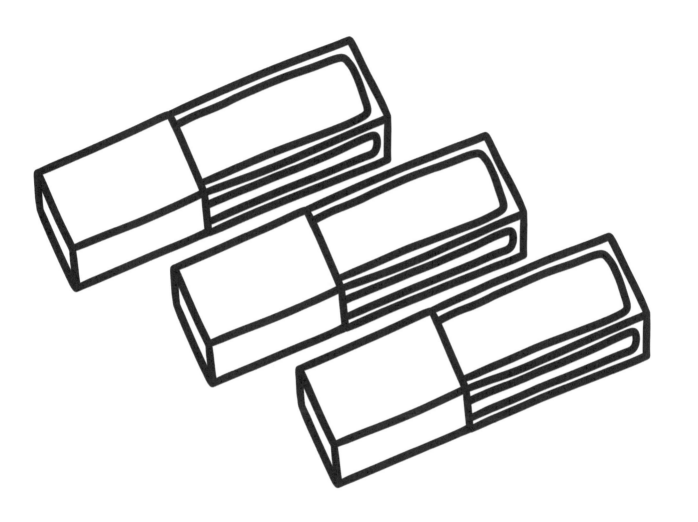

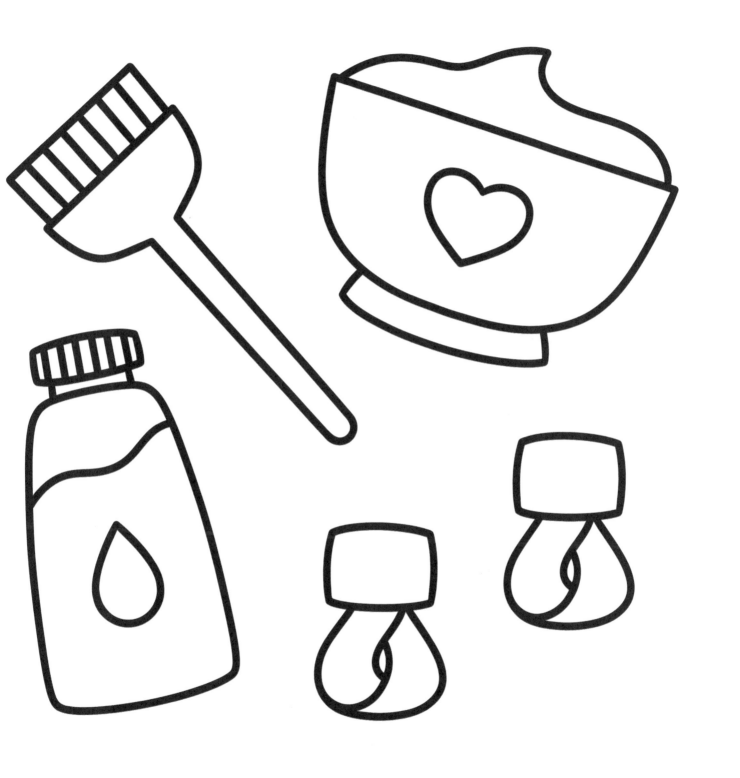

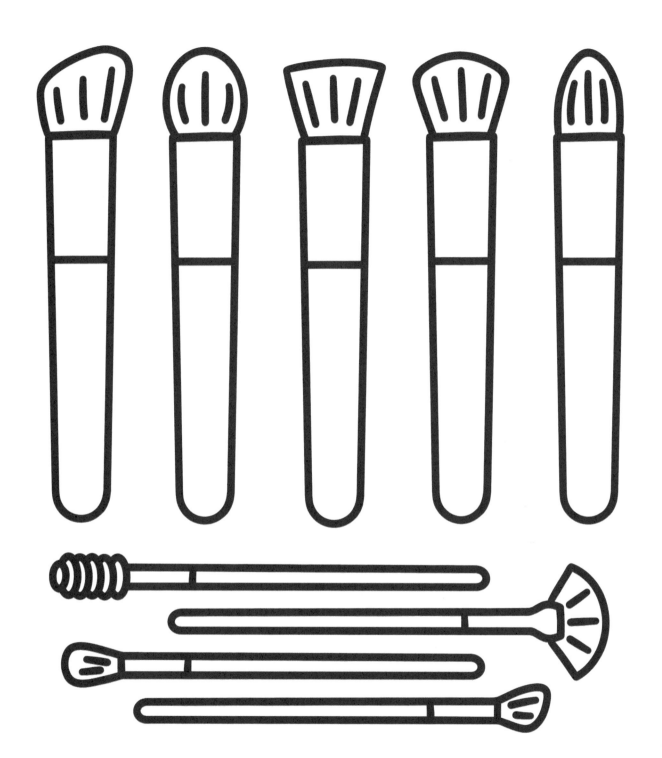

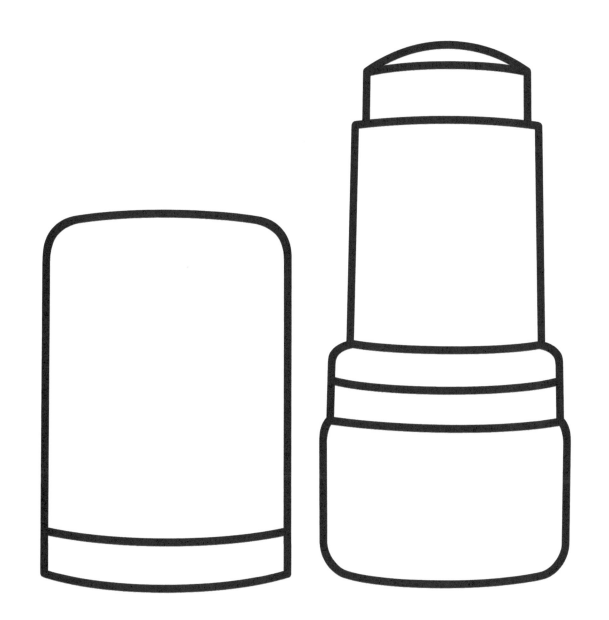

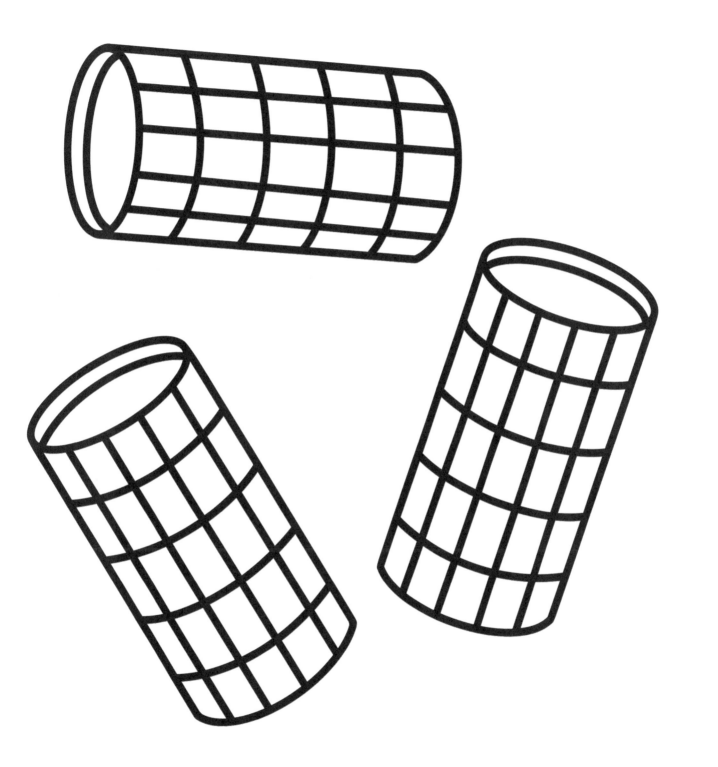

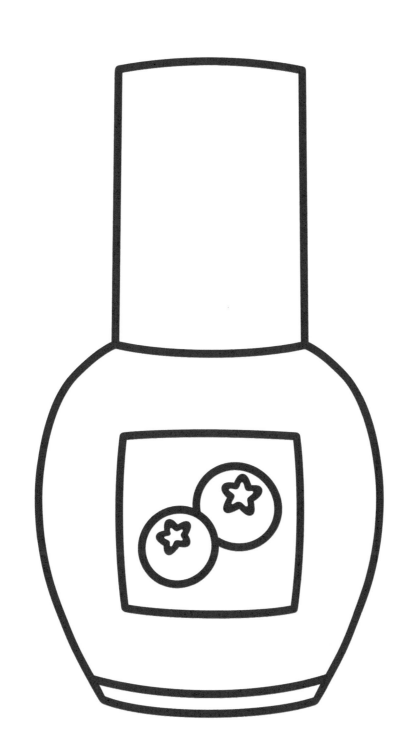

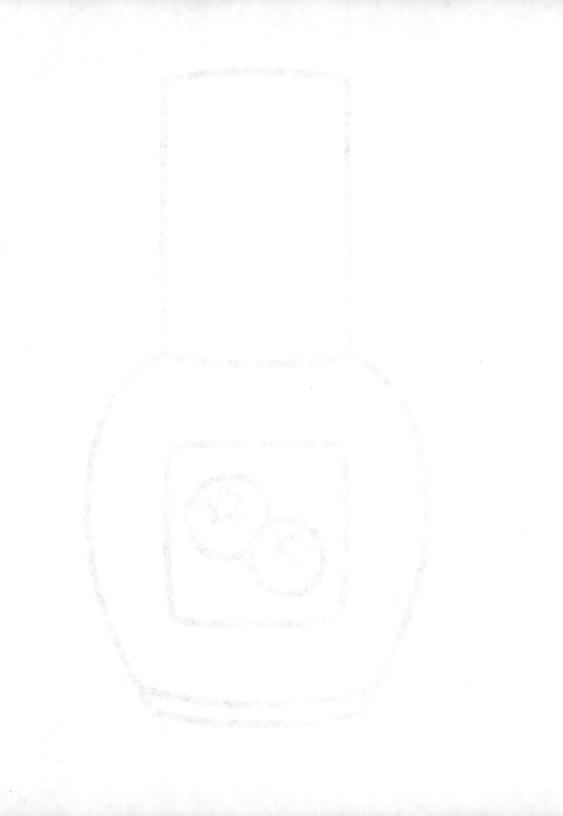

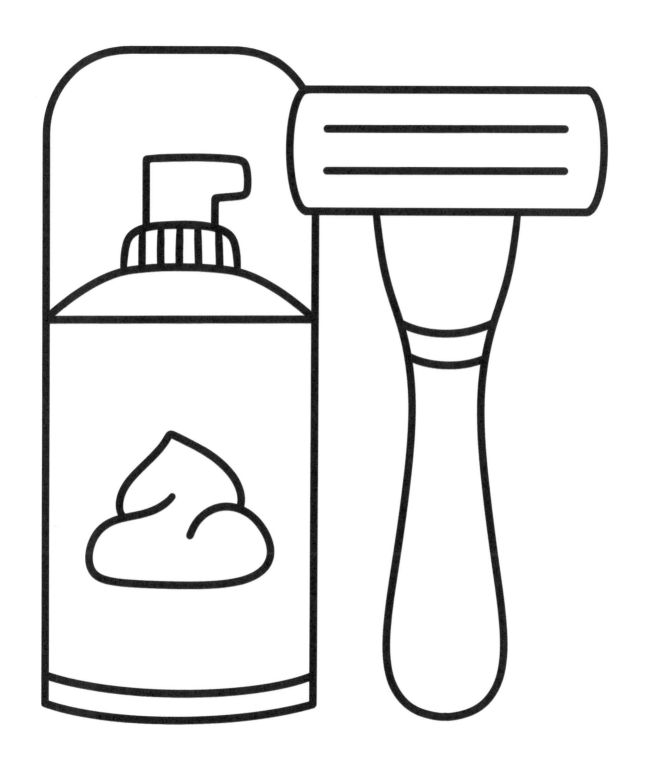

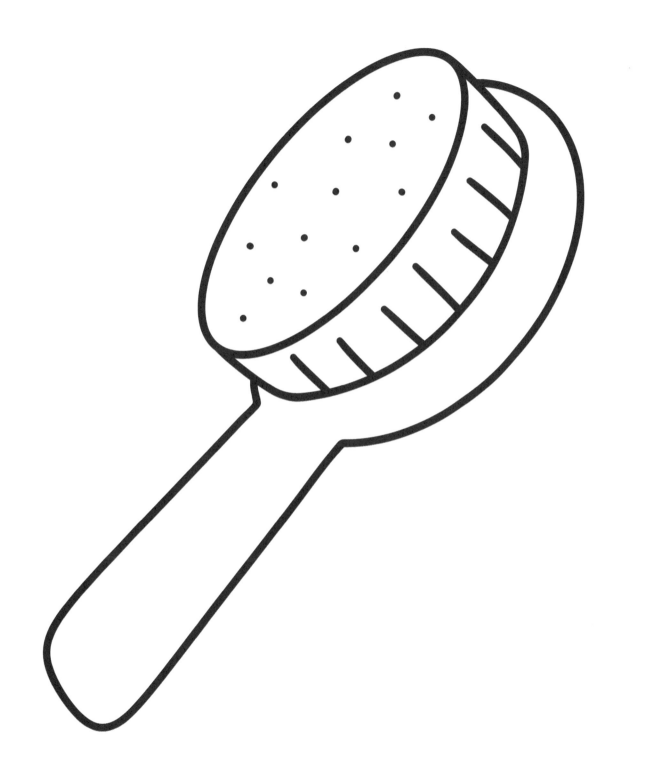

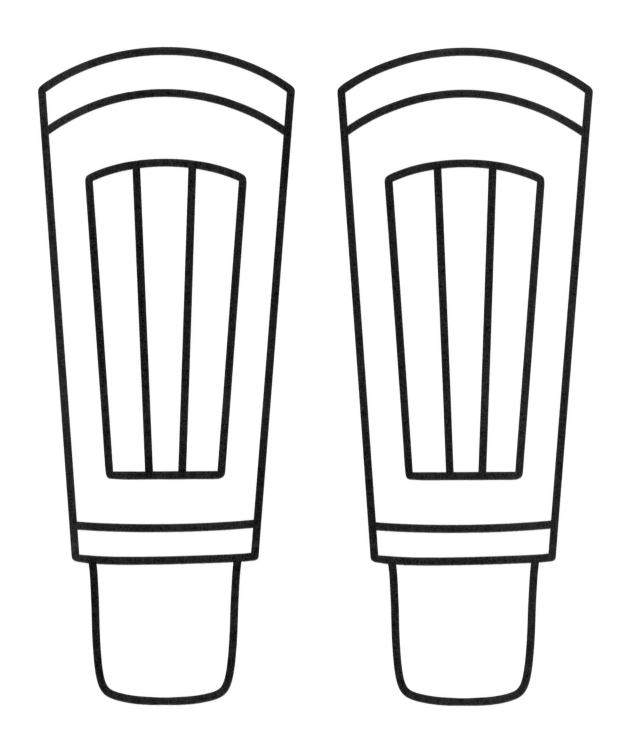

Made in United States
Troutdale, OR
09/25/2024

23134867R00060